Praise for "Poetic Medicine"

Poetic Medicine in the Time of Pandemic offers us a healing tapestry of voices that light our way as we navigate through the maze of this new and foreign world of Covid-19. Hear the poetic songs of fear, isolation, and loss singing, and as we recognize our own voices that perhaps we've held inside, we are joined by a chorus that includes humor and hope. We come to accept the uncertainty of this new planet we all live on together, learning to tend to each new feeling as it arises and find the possibility of growth it offers, no matter where we're planted or what the conditions. Through some of these poems, we learn to sit with ourselves in this current life-pause, noticing the glories around us, the small things we used to take for granted that now give us joy and hope. *Poetic Medicine* should be read one or two poems at a time, like spoonfuls of bitters, a prescription written by a doctor of heart and spirit, to help us metabolize, heal, and have courage in this new life where we now find ourselves.

— MEREDITH HELLER, MA
    poet and author of *Songlines* and *Write A Poem,*
    and her new book, *Save Your Life,* will be published in 2021

This is an insightful book that advances our collective understanding of the psychological impact that the Covid-19 pandemic has had on the world.

— SAIDA ERRADI, PH.D.
    faculty member, John Hopkins University

Poetic Medicine in the Time of Pandemic is a mirror and a healing balm. Many of the poems address the uncertainty and brokenness that reminds us that we are in this together. It is a heartening reminder of the alchemy that poets use to both hold and heal. Seeing the world as the poets see it allows us to borrow their eyes and remember the world is both smaller and bigger during our shared quarantine. These poems give us space for our anger, our fear, our gratitude, our hope and our imagining the path ahead. Dawn Li has truly given us healing medicine in this lovely collection.

   —Wendi R. Kaplan
     Poet Laureate, Alexandria, Virginia (2016–2019)

The editor compiles moving poems in the spirit of "Love the life we live, live the life we love." In the face of unexpected disasters, poets compassionately offer comfort from the back of the moon, from the eagle's eyes, from high-rise buildings in Manhattan, or in the eyes of masked faces standing six feet away. Behind shut-down windows, poets still see the sun, the moon, and the stars, feel the spring breeze brush their faces, and hear Italians singing from their balconies. The book broadcasts an affectionate melody, gently tugging on our heartstrings. We are not alone in this crisis, as the whole world is in it together. We recall the beauty of the past and we know how to cherish it—even if it's just an early morning cup of Starbucks coffee. One day, we will be free again, and together our spirits will be renewed!

   —Mingming Cheung
     retired interior designer, painter, Founder and CEO of
     Chinese Culture and Art League, Washington, DC

Poetic Medicine in the Time of Pandemic

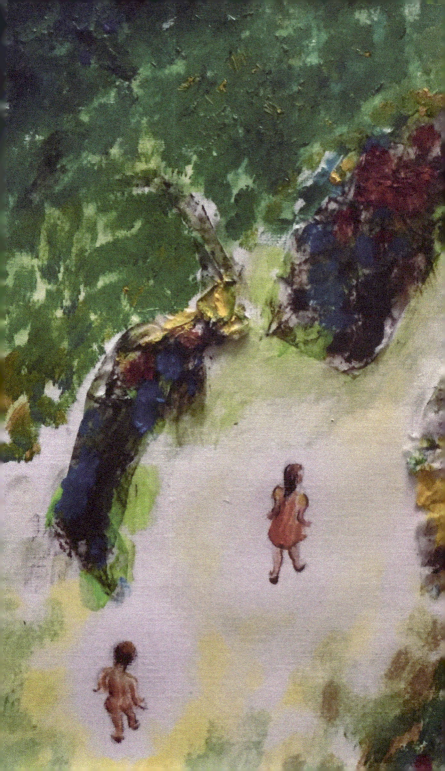

Poetic Medicine
IN THE
Time *of* Pandemic

*A Collection of
Poems from
Around the World*

Edited by Dawn Li, Ph.D.

Paula Goodman, Jon Von Erb,
Jude-brail Umahi, and Frank Leibold, Ph.D.

Illustrated by Yanfang, Ph.D.

PRECOCITY PRESS

Copyright 2020 by Lotus Leaf LLC. All Rights Reserved. Poets and artists retain the copyright of their individual work.

Managing Editor: Dawn Li, Ph.D.
Editor: Brijit Reed
Creative Director and Designer: Susan Shankin
Illustrator: Yanfang, Ph.D.

No part of this book may be reproduced or transmitted in any form or by any means, electronic or mechanical, including photocopying, recording, or by an information storage and retrieval system—except by a reviewer who may quote brief passages in a review to be printed in a magazine, newspaper, or on the web—without permission in writing from the publisher. For permission requests, email the publisher at: susan@precocitypress.com

ISBN: 978-1-7362174-2-9

Published by Precocity Press
Venice, CA 90291

First edition. Printed and bound in the United States of America

For more information, visit poeticmedicinebook.com

TO HUMANITY—

*especially the essential workers
of the global Covid-19 crisis*

CONTENTS

Letter from the Managing Editor	xi
Observations from the Psychologist	xv
Covid-19 Resources	xvii

1. UNCERTAINTY — 1

A Voice for the Broken | Renhui	2
Electric | Anna-Maria Hartner	4
The Matrix | Essama Chiba	6
History Lessons | Kim Escobar	7
How Dare Angels Sing Dark Songs | Sharon Flynn	8
The Ball … | Yanfang	9
The Trouble with Touch | Greg Gaul	10
Mother Earth's Prescription | Paula Goodman	12
The Drive-thru at Starbucks | Kim Escobar	15
Carpe Noctem | Jon Welsh	16
Covid Ovid | Michael McGibney Whelan	18
A World on Pause | Robert Stone	21

2. CONFINEMENT — 23

Love in the Times of Corona | Thanisha Santhosh	24
Doing Nothing | Henrique Formigoni Morais	28

Depression | Glenn Merrilees	30
Be Prepared | Debra Sue Lynn	32
On the Far Side of the Moon | Bobbie Breden	34
Kairos | Henrique Formigoni Morais	35
From Lockdown Windows | Brian Carlin	36
I Have Witnessed | Cecelia Cran	37
I Still Cannot Walk on the Street in May | Peng (Gary) Fang	38
Drizzling | Kim Escobar	40
Consolation | Devon Brock	42
Six Feet Six Feet | Caren Krutsinger	43
Walking the Dog | Jon Welsh	44
Just Want to Stay Away from You | Renhui	46

3. EMBROILED — 47

Working the Front-Lines | Paul Brothers	48
Who Was That Unmasked Man? | Brian Carlin	49
Love Welling Up Inside | Carmela Patterson-Mooney	50
P.E.A.C.E. | Alfred Vassallo	51
See Us Rise | Norbert James	52
I am Waiting | Jianxun Gao	54
The Crone | Olivia Avery	56
My Dragon-Well Sword | Jianxun Gao	59

Evolving | Olivia Avery	60
Poets Making Spiritual Medicine | Renhui	62

4. MOURNING — 65

Shooting Star | Jon Welsh	66
Breathe | Jude-brail Umahi	67
On Passing | Thanisha Santhosh	68
Unmasked | Frank Leibold	70
The Maple | Devon Brock	71
Time for Tears | Paula Goodman	72
At the End of April | Nigel DE Costa	74
Hope Beyond Corona | John Finkelstein	76
My Simple Dream | Archie Haynes	78
Toroidal Healing | Randall S.	80
Endurance | Paula Goodman	82

5. QUEST — 85

Hum | Brijit Reed	86
This is My Prayer | Sarita Verma	88
Healing in the Wind | Jude-brail Umahi	89
Heal Your Wounds | Rowan Vanskyver Killian	90
Pain | Miao Xi	91
A String of Hope | Mythri Arjun	92
The Sparrow's Song | MJ Donnelly	93

As Soldiers of Togetherness, We Win! | Jon Von Erb	94
Rooted | Brijit Reed	96
The True Self | Patricia Rooks	99
Circles of Harmony | Renhui	100
Bird's-Eye View from Under an Oak Tree | Qihong (Richard) Wang	103

6. EMERGING — 105

Nest | Devon Brock	106
Dance Again | Jude-brail Umahi	107
Fellowship | Frank Leibold	108
There is Hope | Aurum di Angelo	109
Here and Now | Thanisha Santhosh	110
This Moment After Covid | Jayantee Khare	115
Wings of Faith | Jude-brail Umahi	116
There's a Seed for Every Sorrow | Fay Ballerino	117
A Flight of Fancy | Phoenix Aradia	118
With the Help of Faith in the Aftermath of Covid-19 | Jon Von Erb	120
Rise | Jude-brail Umahi	122
Acknowledgments	125
Key Contributors	127
Biographies	133

LETTER FROM THE MANAGING EDITOR

WHEN I VISITED my birth country of China in late January of 2020, I was so saddened by what I saw there. The beautiful city of Wuhan, where I spent my formative years, was turned into hellish grounds in the fight to save coronavirus patients. Thousands of Chinese had been thrust into the ongoing tragedy of the deadly coronavirus. When I returned to Washington DC, I wrote my first virus-related poem and posted it on allpoetry.com. As the initial cases were reported in Italy, Spain, and the US (my adopted country), I realized that it was just a matter of time before the coronavirus would hit the whole world, turning everything upside down.

I had to do something. *We had to do something.* Poetry has been used as a powerful healing tool for centuries and has even lifted me from the depths of my own suffering. I had recently published a collection of my poems, *Song Of A Lotus Leaf,* a "memoir" in poetry of the last twenty years of my life. Strung together, these poems had become, for me, stepping stones in the torrential river of my spiritual awakening. It occurred to me that a collection of poems from writers around the world might also have a healing effect on the collective soul of the human race.

Since allpoetry.com is a group of international poets who write about anything and everything that affects our daily lives, that was the first place I turned to for inspiration. Why not mobilize this creative force to offer words of comfort, hope, and wisdom for all?

Poets, Frank Leibold, Jon Von Erb, Jude-brail Umahi, and Paula Goodman immediately joined the effort and emerged as leaders of the group. We ran contests on allpoetry.com with specific themes. College graduate, Yasmeen McGettrick, and graduate student, Jocelyn Zhao, helped gather poems and coordinate meetings. Susan Shankin at Precocity Press immediately endorsed the idea and started brainstorming creative ideas with the team. Within a month, we had collected over 100 poems. Many poets were excited about the effort and offered the use of their writing for free. We were touched by their heartfelt work and their enthusiasm. Brijit Reed later became involved as the manuscript's editor and she identified more new talent from other sources to bring to the project. During this time, a few of us and some of our family members fell sick to the virus, but on we marched.

As we read each poem, a pattern began to emerge from them, leading us down a path of shell shock, struggle, quest, and finally, acceptance and rebirth. This revealed the order in which the poems themselves were to be organized in this text. The concept developed further as we were collecting quotes for the book. We came across many wise sayings from ancient cultures and past poets. Rumi's quote

"The wound is the place where the light enters you," for example, is so true and beautifully put. The wound, be it physical or mental, has matured into pillars of spirituality in our human civilization. Jesus Christ was executed on the cross and came back to save humanity, and the historical Buddha, Shakyamuni, awakened in order to teach others to see that the path for enlightenment is first recognizing that life is suffering.

Since this is a collection of compositions by people around the globe, many of these works are written in the colloquial speech patterns and vocabularies of the poets' homelands and are not specific to any one group or culture. Instead of detracting from the overall message, it reminds us that we're all in this together, providing a sense of immediacy and intimacy, and although some of the poems have been edited for clarity, they are each a valued contribution to our effort. The world is indeed so much smaller than it seems.

I hope this collection of poems, like a bouquet of flowers, offers you solace and beauty, accompanying you through difficult days in this unprecedented time of pandemic. When you feel down, pick it up, and be inspired!

— Dawn Li, Ph.D.
Managing Editor

OBSERVATIONS FROM THE PSYCHOLOGIST

JANUARY 2020 AWAKENED with the optimistic promise that accompanies each New Year. Little did we know that a new virus first identified in Wuhan, China, would soon immobilize and devastate people all over the world. This global pandemic has produced massive anxiety as we've struggled to protect ourselves from a highly contagious but confusing invader that has resulted in nearly a million deaths as of this writing, and left many more people coping with ongoing medical problems, emotional crises, and economic devastation. The world's people have been advised to stay home, wear masks, and be socially distant — all in an effort to curtail this monster that we are valiantly trying to understand and control. Our economies and our lives have been turned upside down, and the great unknown is when, if ever, we will return to some level of normalcy. 2020 is a defining time for these living generations — and our world will be forever changed by its ramifications.

In response to this time of pain and tumult, a group of poets, organized by Dr. Dawn Li, have come together from around the world to share the powers of poetic healing. Jon Von Erb, Frank Leibold, Paula Goodman, and many others have generously contributed their time and talent for the creation of this book. Throughout the years, poetry has provided an avenue for sharing stories about our feelings during these struggles — how we are not alone in our strife, the various paths we can take toward finding strength in ourselves, and the inspiration that can help us weather the storms that are inevitably part of life. *Poetic Medicine* cannot heal all ills, but this small book draws on the power of poetry to help make us feel stronger, less isolated, and more whole while we are engaged in this pandemic odyssey together.

We recognize that the stresses in coping with our pandemic world will exacerbate old emotional issues while instigating serious anxiety and depression in others. Please seek mental health treatment if you are experiencing:

- persistent anxiety or depression for most of the day over a 2–week period
- changes in sleep or eating patterns
- persistent difficulty in sleeping, concentrating, or making decisions
- heightened irritability, causing angry outbursts toward family members
- increased smoking, alcohol, or other drug consumption

With the advent of telehealth, obtaining help is easier and more available than ever.

—JEANNE M. BOLTON, PH.D.

Dr. Bolton has been in private practice in Columbia, MD, for over 30 years, specializing in treatment of depression and anxiety disorders, with particular emphasis on stress and medical disorders.

COVID-19 RESOURCES

The Center for Disease Control and Prevention (CDC) has a great deal of helpful information listed on their website, which is presented here to help encourage you to get help, if needed.

- Call 911
- Substance Abuse and Mental Health Services Administration Disaster Distress Helpline (samhsa.gov/disaster-preparedness): 1-800-985-5990 (press 2 for Spanish), or text "TalkWithUs" for English or "Hablanos" for Spanish to 66746. Spanish speakers from Puerto Rico can text "Hablanos" to 1-787-339-2663
- Substance Abuse and Mental Health Services Administration's National Helpline (samhsa.gov/find-help/national-helpline): 1-800-662-HELP (4357) and TTY 1-800-487-4889
- Treatment Services Locator (findtreatment.samhsa.gov)
- National Suicide Prevention Lifeline (suicidepreventionlifeline.org): 1-800-273-TALK (8255) for English, 1-888-628-9454 for Spanish, or Lifeline Crisis Chat (suicidepreventionlifeline.org/chat).
- National Domestic Violence Hotline (thehotline.org): 1-800-799-7233 or text "LOVEIS" to 22522
- National Child Abuse Hotline (childhelp.org/hotline): 1-800-4AChild (1-800-422-4453) or text 1-800-422-4453
- National Sexual Assault Hotline 1-800-656-HOPE (4673) or Online Chat (hotline.rainn.org/online)
- The Eldercare Locator (eldercare.acl.gov/Public/Index.aspx): 1-800-677-1116 TTY Instructions (eldercare.acl.gov/public/about/contact_Info/Index.aspx) or email Eldercare Locator at eldercarelocator@n4a.org
- Veteran's Crisis Line (veteranscrisisline.net/): 1-800-273-TALK (8255) or Crisis Chat (veteranscrisisline.net/get-help/chat) or text: 8388255. Resources for deaf and hard of hearing: 1-800-799-4889
- LGBT National Help Center (glbthotline.org/): 888-843-4564

1 UNCERTAINTY

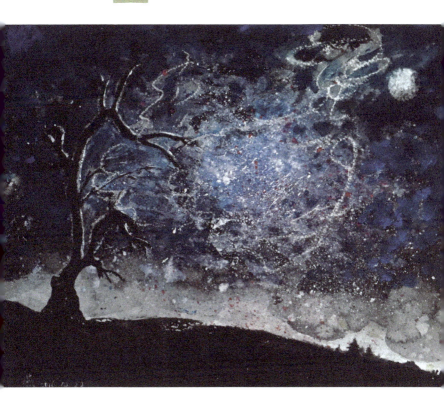

True wisdom comes to each of us when we realize how little we understand about life, ourselves, and the world around us.

—SOCRATES

A VOICE FOR THE BROKEN | RENHUI

i was a rose
a blooming
rose

until a wind
across the ocean
struck me

my petals
fell
broken

into drops
of blood
on sand

a poet
saw me

Uncertainty

turned me
into letters —
p
o
e
t
r
y

she took my picture
with her phone
and sent me off

i became
her voice

a voice
for the broken

ELECTRIC | ANNA-MARIA HARTNER

Dear broken self,

You are a polarized light,
a twisted body
in one sleeping lotus,
shaken by Berlin winds
and morning sonatas.

If I had guessed your
touch was arctic,
I would not have built
this glass house —
this midnight city
of wordless poetry —

but we were once spring,
and each day was a promise
carefully wrapped in our
electric hearts.

I beg,
from the rooftop I stand,
do not let loss
nor life
bury you.

Uncertainty

Love,
you are an eternity.

Hold on to that
cinnamon sunrise
and fragile hope,

for I will carry you
to our corner of the
Universe,
to these constellations
and wild things we chase

so that we might awake
to imagine one last
English sky
and stolen moment
in this tattered town
where we now reside.

Love,
your unspoken promises

THE MATRIX | ESSAMA CHIBA

Feeling the depth of days
bearing the weight of time
Countless nights
caught in the matrix

A visual cortex
broken frames
Fields of data
fragmented
sown with glitches

The bitter reap
of emotional malfunction
our hidden pain

Most inner thoughts
on display
in cyberspace
at the edge
of a keyboard

Uncertainty

HISTORY LESSONS | KIM ESCOBAR

I remember salad bars like they might be some exotic relic from the past that I'll tell my grandchildren about/buffets/ frozen yogurt shops where you put your own toppings on/my grandchildren will look at me/eyes wide above their masks/ trying to imagine such a world/

HOW DARE ANGELS SING DARK SONGS | SHARON FLYNN

down in the deepest depths
despair finds a way to grow
silence allows the dark to win
while arrows fly by night
and hit their mark

all the flowers die
leaves wither with no sunlight
silence allows dark angels to steal
every beam of light from frightened hearts

dead streets emptied of feet
masks on faces rob breath and hide smiles
silence allows greed to spin the wheel
while heros have no masks to keep them safe

how dare angels sing dark themes
and tell their blatant lies to the masses
silence sits on the truth until it expires
no rescue planned, opiate lies
crammed down our throats

quarantined, trapped like rats
nowhere to run, angels sing of death
silence keeps us chained to fear
a phone call unlocks silence, awakens
soul rivers to rise up, waters to heal

THE BALL . . . | YANFANG

A boy kicked the ball far and high
and the red ball fell asleep because it was tired.
A girl knocked over a bottle of blue ink,
and smeared it over earth and sky.
The cat fell in love with the ball,
but the jealous ink restrained the cat.
Breasts swelled and longing opened,
in a dream of blue, red, and white.

But a black Greed jumping to the roof,
a yellow Pride haunting down the stairs below,
a red Virus staring into Man defies,
with her mortal taste bringing only woe.
Time to remember Heaven and Earth Rising from Chaos.
Time to search Oracle of God from Siloa's brook.
Time to praise all the Heroes from Aonian Mount
Ahead, the blue eternity is hoisting the Red Hope!

THE TROUBLE WITH TOUCH | GREG GAUL

The trouble with touch
is wanting too much
Fingertips that tingle
Trite hearts, good signal

Your space in-between
where feelings are seen
If taken one day
you lose your way

The rush of desire
an embrace on fire
Sparks of connection
human convection

As all isolate
Some suffer cruel fate
More virus distress
of touchless duress

Uncertainty

Sharing a fresh start
by staying apart
Resisting to touch
now saves lives as such

Distancing does work
recovery shall perk
Resources will align
when all forces combine

The best way to touch
comes through in the clutch
When all's said and done
our world can be one

MOTHER EARTH'S PRESCRIPTION | PAULA GOODMAN

Is Mother Earth now crying
or have we been denying
that her tears were flowing
For so long she was showing

all the signs we cannot see
We're not checking reality
What is happening to all of us
It's too late when we fuss

Her pain started when
the earth was full of sin
There is goodness to see too
It is our Mother's faithful virtue

Was she born or did she always exist
Do we settle just to subsist
What part do we have to play
when Dear Mother has to pay

She has planted and conducted
All she gave to us instructed
Underneath our marching feet
Mother Earth and her heartbeat

Mass corruption and dispute
Nature's arms, we refute
Something here is amiss
Look around at all of this

Every part of every land
She does love and understand
all her children, nature too
Now she cries over you

Don't you think it's time to turn
Look at her and really learn
that what we need and what we want
becomes a nightmare she will haunt

In order to find an answer here
we need our Mother Earth so dear
All the beauty she has given
for us to love and keep on living

We have somehow redirected
Everything now is just so hectic
When her breath became the fire
Mother's tears showed her desire

To the oceans her tears fell
and tried to clear the plastic well
Her eyes, the sun, where she is light
Her soul, of course, the core delight

Mother Earth to us is telling
look around and stop the yelling
It doesn't matter where you are
if you look she'll show her scar

When we ignore the purest tears
we become our biggest fears
What we hide does manifest
The illness is now addressed

Oh, the symptoms and description
Mother Earth has the prescription
All the steps of all her children
we walk upon her penicillin

Take stock of what she has offered
More than you she has suffered
There is a way to help her live
only if we learn to give.

Uncertainty

THE DRIVE-THRU AT STARBUCKS | KIM ESCOBAR

i'm at the drive-thru at starbucks/and i order a caramel spice latte/just because i like the sound of it/and it doesn't really matter what i get/you ask for an orange juice and a bagel/and we drive out of there/and i didn't think about it/ but i must've thought life might always be that simple/we didn't know then that pandemics could happen in our lifetime/ people we loved would die/others would struggle/illness would come our way/we knew, even then, our biggest decisions weren't at Starbucks/but we didn't know how big they would become/

CARPE NOCTEM | JON WELSH

*Now seize the night; embrace death
as passionately as life, as flowers' beauty
precedes fate, cut or moldering,
feeding generations.*

*We flower, opening with light
and lingering until darkness comes
creeping upon us. Or not so gently
as to come unimplored in sleep;
the catastrophes of birth and death
mingle incestuously, make us crazy
with mortality and its fearsome remedy.*

*Remind me –
perhaps I will remember you if we meet,
if we meet again in a different circumstance.
I struggle to remember myself
moment to moment, losing others,
chasing who I am while pursuing you.*

Uncertainty

Thus the danger of the other, even oneself;
pursuit is a dangerous expedition.
We seized this, and now find ourselves
here, unless you're lost, absent,
drunk with thought
whose mysteries of logic
stupefy faith.

So says the tree that grows
where soil lies fallow
and seed seldom takes root.

COVID OVID | MICHAEL MCGIBNEY WHELAN

Welcome
to the crasher party of
Covid Ovid
Century 21's mega meta of
morphosis

It marched in on us in March
like Nazis into Paris
conquering the world we once presumed
a takeforgranted given
sudden outanowhere shape
shifted in the flick
of a few days round
St. Paddy's Day

All now gone
Yeats
Echoes of Easter 1916: ALL
is
 "changed
        changed utterly"

into a new utterness
avatared
into
an alien sadist morpher

whose Joker touch turns

Uncertainty

innocent everydaytouch into
Pariah Touch of
sudden henceforth

    touch

        un-

            welcome

        un-

            safe

Leaving each me of we
trans-
    figured
        into
            strangers
to be
exigent exiled
from me and from
every other in the we
who once was a WE

gonged game-changed
riding in a daily roll wheeling in
a new Russian Covid roulette:
my life/my death vs
their lives/their deaths —
latest looser count: 225K USA

I/You so-far-maybe-safe-escaped
but hostaged still by breath threats
riding unmasked invisible
in iddybiddy aerosoled
muthfuka breath bubbles of molecules
hijacking
coughs
    and sneezes
        and innocent
            choral voices in song

lung hunting
    blood vein seeking
        micro gadding
in tacky
    particle-spiked coronas

            killable only
by an irony
    of soap and wipes—
        and

d.
  i.
    s.
      t.
        a.
          n.
c.
  e.

A WORLD ON PAUSE | ROBERT STONE

a world on pause,
and we witness ourselves in truth.

inside is always scary —
four walls and some furniture
a few apertures for vitamin d,
moments captured in snapshots,
captioned "quarantine life."
captioned "pandemic 2020."

inside is scarier when you're inside already.
nowhere to look but at an imprisoned body;
a soul twisted, gnarled, and knotty;
a mind fuzzy with liquor; a memory spotty.

we go stir-crazy in isolation,
clutching a fur baby for support.
i've been hurt lately.
i've been curt lately.
i voted to let the virus run its course.

a world on pause,
and we deny every shade of our truth.

2 CONFINEMENT

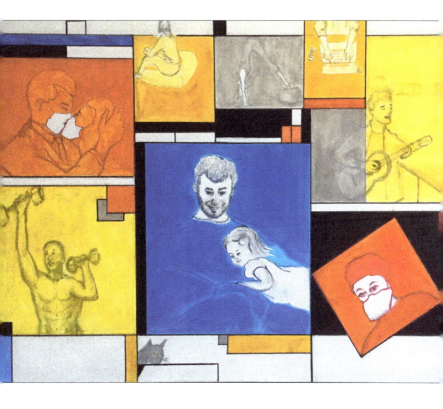

Knowing others is intelligence;
knowing yourself is true wisdom.
Mastering others is strength;
mastering yourself is true power.
—LAO TZU

LOVE IN THE TIMES OF CORONA | THANISHA SANTHOSH

After the government told us
that we were no longer to leave the house,
and after a month's worth of quarrels
between us; often about
what to watch on TV or the color
of my cotton blouse on our weekly trip
to the supermarket or the lack of sugar
in the hibiscus tea,
my lover and i decided the world
was in dire need of kindness,
starting with us,
and that perhaps language was a great place to begin.

We no longer term our bickering as a fight
(he corrects me and calls it a
minor misunderstanding).
To make matters better and because
we are both rather docile as far as animals go,
I smile and nod and tell him
he is right,
that our anger (corrected : misplaced passion)
must be diluted from sediment —
into something more yielding;
and because we declare our love to be tender —
deer's nose / boiled carrots / salt soaked lamb meat /
the pulpy gap left behind by fallen milk teeth . . .

Because we declare our love to be
not only tender but also enormous,
like the soft boiled egg of an ostrich or
a tranquillised elephant that has just had
its tusk pulled out,
we decide
that the nomenclature of our love
will have no place for vindictive words.

We spend the afternoon
with our spines bent over dictionaries,
blackening out and then replacing
astringent words we might use as weapons.
Our vernacular will now no longer include
words like hurt *or* heartache.
Instead, we will say
i am yearning for your kindness.

Distrust *is now redundant*
and so is doubt;
instead, we will apologise
for a vacillating heart,
although
morally *inconspicuous, it will be a*
more severe but accepted replacement.

We do away with blame, resent;
strike out enraged, incandescent;
leave no room for malevolence
to bloom.
Instead of heartburn *we will say*
come hear this choleric call of my viscera,
the past *will now be called*
an incessant *cloying*
or that which we no longer paint with words
(best to leave some lingo behind).

A word like hostility *makes way for*
I wish you would hold me
but I'm too proud to ask.
Hot temper *is renamed a* momentary malady
of the mind
and arguments *will now be called*
debates for the downcast.

Of course it is not simple to ease into
this new argot
and so we grant ourselves two weeks
to make a smooth transition.
Until then, all sentences must end
with love *or* beloved *or an equally affectionate*
synonym.

Confinement

Sarcasm is, of course, allowed
in degrees that are not vitriolic
and as long as it always leads
to lovemaking,
and touching is to be greatly increased
in both quantity
and urgency.

We spend the afternoon making a litmus test, of sorts,
testing the acidity of our new words.
When we are pleased we lay belly to belly
on the floor and touch,
counting on two sets of fingers
twelve-hundred odd words transformed
into tenderness.

Of course, there are still some nasty words
for which we could find no suitable replacement.
To avoid using them, at all costs,
when their need arises
in heated conversations
we have decided, instead, to kiss
until our gums bleed.

DOING NOTHING | HENRIQUE FORMIGONI MORAIS

Sometimes it's worth doing nothing
at all. Life isn't just about the chores
that buzz and fly around our heads,
but that we know. What you perhaps don't
realise is that the vacation of your lifetime
or weaving a masterpiece
or falling in love aren't all that matter either.
Sometimes it's good to just sit
between the four walls of the body
while the world stretches and fades
over its own memory,
like the yellow streetlight, when
it blows through your window in the wee hours.
I'm not talking about watching television
as it drains time from you through
the tubes they use for transfusing blood
while you lie on the sofa, drooling and emptying.

Confinement

Doing nothing isn't wasting time.
Opening the kitchen sink
to watch the water bend and curl
and figure out its waterness
isn't a waste of water.
Take a seat and enjoy doing nothing. Look closely
as the fallen leaves sink into the ground.
Pace around the room in pilgrimage.
Read your skin as it wrinkles in the mirror.
Glue your head to the pillow
and close your eyes without falling asleep,
submerged in silence.

DEPRESSION | GLENN MERRILEES

see me through the darkness
see me through the gloom
depression made a home for me
a cell, a tiny room

reaching out for answers
I try to quell the pain
someone stole my sunshine
I'm in the dark again

there's loved-ones all around me
arms stretched out in aid
depression's grips are stronger
it's me who's being played

thoughts come to haunt me
keep flashing through my head
you useless waste of time
I'd feel better if you're dead

Confinement

*I'm just a sinking battleship
on a stormy sea of pain
a jellyfish upon a beach
beneath an acid rain*

*this sickness keeps returning
on and off for years
I've fought so many battles
I've shed so many tears*

*yet I shall keep on fighting
as I have no other choice
ignoring all this madness
and that suicidal voice*

*so listen here depression
put this upon your wall
I'll crush you under my heel
and I shall stand up tall*

BE PREPARED | DEBRA SUE LYNN

*Be prepared! Sufficient supplies of necessaries should
be kept: medicines, paper products, stores of food—non-
perishables, dry milk, plenty of water, salt, cleaning items.
Everything that could sustain you for two weeks or longer.*

*Consider if we lost electric and power: we'll need dry staples,
boxed or in cans. Learn to ration—toilet paper is wasteful.
Practice new methods of sanitizing and cleansing.
We must learn to conserve and contemplate ample
flashlights and batteries.*

*Perhaps include an outdoor camping stove and sufficient
means for cooling medicines that must be refrigerated, or
they will perish. Also be certain you have a non-electric
can opener that works well, and paper plates could be
useful if water supply is low. Several coolers*

*have ice packs for necessary items to be preserved.
Cell phones charged, blankets packed. Have the mind-set
of a serious camper ready for emergencies. Keep ample
funds in cash available, be sure your bills have been kept
up to date, and automobile gas tanks filled and in*

good running condition. Have a means of outside communication should telephones and computers go down—i.e., a battery-operated radio with power to regenerate itself. Have ample trash bags and trash container. If city garbage is stopped, they will contain

*your waste. We must learn to conserve by eating less, wasting less, spending less on non-essentials, and spending more for sustainable products. Always keep disinfectants handy, like hand-wipes.
Utilize your thought*

*processes. Economize. Stay away from places and people who could contaminate you and your loved ones.
Be intelligent and above all else, stay calm. Panic and worry will not serve you! Be prepared. Be safe. Stay well.*

ON THE FAR SIDE OF THE MOON | BOBBIE BREDEN

No others on this moon,
I stay to myself.
My meals are simple—
packages from a shelf.

I stay in my domain,
it's safer in here.
If I venture out,
I'm in protective gear.

The outside is hostile,
a danger to my health.
Too much trauma out there,
but in here, there's health.

With details of my mission
I'm at ease in my brain.
As long as I'm protected,
I've little to complain.

I hope to return
to my home planet soon.
Who knew there'd be so much light
on the far side of the moon?

KAIROS | HENRIQUE FORMIGONI MORAIS

The sun crawls down the belly of the world,
and a day-sweated linen shirt falls from my body,
icicles touched by spring.
Curled stone foeti, bitter in its mineral sleep.
Hands unblossom, seizing the heart.
The heart herself wrapped in the flesh of the breast,
like the light of the furnace wrapping the bread.
Coals grow cold from the inside out.
A moth flickers, clipped by the dark.
The bodies on the newspaper,
knots of rigor mortis undone, fade away.
Their blood, a twilight.
Let this world unpeel from your skin,
fall from you like the consummation cloak.
Let this poem harden into a memory,
its words an oxidizing nonsense.
Jigsaw puzzles unmade without regret,
plastic pieces scattered on the carpet floor.
Hide back into your box of flowers,
your glass house, your anemone,
while these eyelids, like a tent
or dull amber, fold themselves, huge over you.

FROM LOCKDOWN WINDOWS | BRIAN CARLIN

A murmuration swoops, curls
blackly against creeping dusk
seen silently from indoors.

I imagine the camaraderie in furious wings —
the machinations of large populations
where all are bound in keeping an even distance
and rarely stare a neighbour in the eye.

I don't deny the beauty of it, the collective mind in flight —

but all this is from where I stand,
from lockdown windows,

and not the birds-eye view
of small town minds where
small good mornings
and bare civilities
kept us comfortably apart.

I HAVE WITNESSED | CECELIA CRAN

I have witnessed the flight of the falcon
the startling blue of the jay
have watched by the riverbank
the wild things come to play
I have seen so much
back in my childhood days
now, in lockdown, in my home
I miss those wonderful sights
but thank the Lord for my dreams
where I see them every night

I STILL CANNOT WALK ON THE STREET IN MAY | PENG (GARY) FANG

(1)
Covid has suspended my life—
What May!
I sleep in bed the first day,
wake up dreaming the second day,
lie on the couch the third day,
rock on the balcony the fourth day,
and stare out the window the fifth day...
Cold wind blows through Manhattan,
my soul burns in the alley.
Standing alone on an empty New York street,
only with desolation and misery.

(2)
Desert-like faces,
virus-like stars,
death has come to the weak, to the vulnerable,
and to seniors.
Gaze at the deserted cityscape,
countless pairs of eyes from the windows.
June will come, and the sun will shine.
On Times Square, summer will arrive,
sending the dancing breeze.
We will be free,
walking on the New York streets
like the galloping ocean waves!

DRIZZLING | KIM ESCOBAR

*the mist taps on my window/beckons me
to meet somewhere/like lovers/i open
my window/and am overwhelmed by its
damp embrace/it conjures memories of wet
wool sweaters/and fireside afternoons
wrapped up in blankets and books/the
mist tells me of so many days that have
been/centuries of foggy days/and i fall
into histories/while it insinuates itself
under my skin/branding me/and claiming me/
the dampness is a surcease/a balm to the
tumult/and its quiet beauty/shows me more
than it hides/*

*i step outside/as an escape/from too much
togetherness/and too much of myself/the
rain plays across my skin/hangs like fairy lights
lights in trees/stipples the leaves/
whose faces turn up/awaiting benediction/*

Confinement

*it falls like a cloak about my shoulders/
comforting me/and when I look up/to feel
the rain on my face/i see each drop/as if
they are snowflakes/and yet/they fall as
one/choreographed/like a ballet/*

*i see myself reflected in the drops/and i
want to fall with them/be a mere reflection/
of who i was before/*

*this one corner feels remote/the chaos of
new rules and new words/distant/the rain
washes the world clean/and for just a
moment/it doesn't exist/*

CONSOLATION | DEVON BROCK

Out,
beyond the reflection
of yellow kitchen walls,
the green couch and the black dog,
nose prints, tulips, and daylilies
break soil along the driveway.
I not so much see as know.

The first finch grips the strut
of an empty feeder, and the chimes
lament a minor tune. Certainly,
robins gather winterfall and
warblers crest the gulf, and soon,
perhaps, move on.

But for now, I am
content to tap a window
and wait. For later,
when the fever breaks,
and we emerge
into full green summer.

The fledgling will have fledged,
fruits will be well nigh plumped,
and we'll taste summer
as if for the first time.

SIX FEET SIX FEET | CAREN KRUTSINGER

Bonnie calls me to complain
about an insane person
who was yelling, "Six feet! Six feet!" at her
in the grocery store.
Bonnie wears neither masks nor gloves.
She believes the coronavirus pandemic is a hoax
perpetrated by Democrats and Independents.

My next phone call is from my friend Elise,
a wide-eyed liberal from Missouri.
She is complaining about an insane woman
wearing neither masks or gloves
who was getting too close to her in the grocery store.
"I was yelling, 'Six feet! Six feet!'
and she kept coming," she said.

WALKING THE DOG | JON WELSH

I'm writing poems I can't read
through the tsunami roiling my eyes
while you wonder
what the commotion is all about.
How many tears do you have;
who will cipher them?
Mine come from rainstorms and geysers,
flash floods and storm surges,
from distant storms disturbingly close,
weather we all endure
though many will not acknowledge.
But my dog needs walking,
so here I go. To know me
is to walk with me in the rain
while I return the only love
I know, this furry beast
full of kindness, a friend from another species
who loves me no matter how alien I am.

Confinement

*I thought to bring this up gingerly
but it's not my style, not usually,
though I can be tactful at times.
Politic. I've had some wins,
some losses; I prove
net gain, though less perfect
than I desire to be. Or not.
Desiring God is a disaster; yet
when the kingdom of God is within you
the devil to overcome is yourself.
I have yet to figure out the joy in trees,
the beauty of flowers, the purpose
for microbes, ants, or people.
It lies not in the words of others,
though all words reflect
what we don't understand
even when they explain what we do.*

JUST WANT TO STAY AWAY FROM YOU | RENHUI

Another day of lockdown.
We went for a stroll
at a riverside wildlife preserve.

We put on our masks
his with bubbling beer; mine with yin-yang cats —
we kissed

"Cute! Your cats are
drinking his beer!"
a passer-by laughed.

We saw two eagles on bare branches
watched beavers swim
and a group of geese fly over an eyot.

Two women on the roadside looked up
"What are you looking at?"
"Nothing. Just want to stay away from you,"
they said, as 6-feet away they passed.

3 EMBROILED

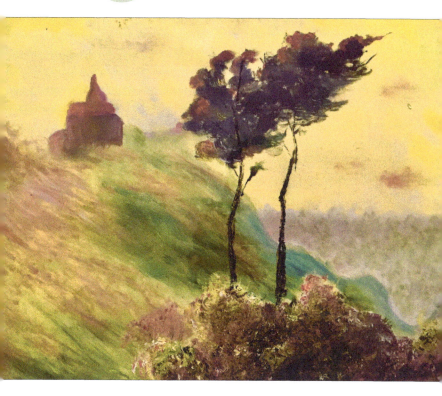

*How many desolate creatures on the earth
have learnt the simple dues of fellowship and
social comfort, in a hospital."*

—ELIZABETH BARRET BROWNING

WORKING THE FRONT-LINES | PAUL BROTHERS

Susan entered ICU, donning both mask and gown,
gloved each of her hands, first left and then right
She took a deep breath, her mask hiding her frown.

A nearby nurse yelled, "I need help over here!"
Susan didn't hesitate, she reacted from instinct.
She grabbed the defibrillator, then shouted, "Clear!"

Too little, too late. The patient's pulse faded away.
"Move this one out! Bring that one over here!"
"Have we a ventilator?" She asked with dismay.

The woman couldn't breathe, her gasping routine.
Susan saw a ventilator down the hall.
"Somebody hurry — get that machine!"

They rushed it in to help open the patient's airways.
"I thank you," the woman said to Susan and the others.
It's the first decent breath that she'd had in three days.

Susan left the ICU and took off her gloves and her gown.
Not sure about mask removal, she left the thing on.
She took a deep breath, her mask hiding her frown.

WHO WAS THAT UNMASKED MAN? | BRIAN CARLIN

A tease for the real plague a-coming:
the dearth of food, jobs, and kindnesses.

This feels like the bloody-good-war
I wished on us as punishment for our fat lives,
in my curmudgeon bed, in the wee hours.

Darwin versus the Freedom Evangelists.
If only vicarious stupidity kept its own company.

But coughs and sneezes spread uneases.
And day in, day out of days in are making me smaller.

Now we're all Niqabbed-up
and having assimilated Islam and outed otherness,

we can smirk ruefully at the bare-faced deniers
who bravely put their grandmas on the frontline
but never tell them.

The COVID party which we're all dressed up for
always has somewhere to go.

Yet the streets are full of superheroes,
giving us all a fighting chance.

Who'd've thought the day'd arrive that going to a store
we'd be wary of the unmasked man and what he'd *give you?*

LOVE WELLING UP INSIDE | CARMELA PATTERSON-MOONEY

When I see a person wearing his or her mask
I feel a sense of grateful pride
that the dear person has taken to heart that task
and has taken it all in stride.

As long as we care for one another we will
hope for a better tomorrow.
Our new normal is in following a new drill.
Hindsight's lessons we can borrow

to carry us on to a future that's brighter
for every man, woman, and child.
We can make our brother's load a little lighter
with every need reconciled.

There is hope for every nation worldwide
when we all have love welling up inside.

P.E.A.C.E. | ALFRED VASSALLO

PEOPLE longing for love and not hate,
tranquillity with their friends and families.
Sharing their hopes and giving respect,
with all races eradicating the bigotry disease.

EARNESTNESS stories with love intense,
co-ordinating the many mixed hearts of humans.
Surrendering to empathy for all that it's worth,
for that is the place where social connection begins.

ACCORD with strangers met on our journeys,
on airplanes, trains, automobiles, or walks.
Different tongues, traditions, and cultures,
with friendly toasts and a variety of talks.

CONCILIATION with our worst enemies,
forgetting the eye-for-an-eye notion,
for loving the foe is a much greater love.
In the eyes of God, it is the true devotion.

EXALTATION throughout a peaceful world,
happiness injected into our warm and anxious blood.
Children born to a wonderful life,
forgetting that once our esteem
was truly drowned in COVID-19.

SEE US RISE | NORBERT JAMES

coronavirus knocked and
we opened our doors to the unknown
an uninvited guest who would not leave

it sucked the breath from our neighbors
our frontline workers and our elderly
it frightened us into our sanitized homes

and then our rise became
the Italian singers at sunset from every window
New Yorkers banging pots to honor survivors & dead

children feeding the hungry
grandmas making the masks
coming together to meet the needs of others

controversy and confusion coronavirus sowed
common sense came late to visit, didn't always stay
caring and communication zoomed into the room

Embroiled

don't tells us what to do, just
tell us what needs to be done
let us learn to live with sickness invisibly near

peace to you my brother, my sister, my neighbor, my friend
our neighbor built the sign and hung it on their fence
and I didn't protest, yes all lives matter,
some need more help

and we slog on laboring to the next benchmark
some will not distance, some will not mask,
but the majority care and nurture so we will heal.
See us rise.

I AM WAITING | JIANXUN GAO
(TRANSLATION BY JOCELYN ZHAO, REVISED BY DAWN LI)

At the sound of a chime
I can't help but look at my phone.
Reading WeChat group emails
has become a daily thing.
A few words from you, my dear friend,
offers me the best of company.

Many times silently,
I've read those same emails.
Innocent sayings
send tears to my eyes.
I cry and then laugh.
The seed sown in my heart
grows into a deep longing.

*Don't you see my joy ripple
when you pass by and smile at me?
There are fewer regrets
and more eagerness
this spring.*

*You work in the hospital
in the coronavirus wing
Each time I open our WeChat group
I seem to enter your office.
Face-to-face, we talk and sing.*

*Protect yourself, my darling friend.
For your safe return, I am waiting!*

THE CRONE | OLIVIA AVERY

I am the crone,
silvery hair swirling in the moonlight.
Staff in hand, I stand in my dignity,
a mystic descending through
the mists of time.

I'm here amid the slaughter of millions
by an invisible enemy
that leaves a wake of destruction behind.

A sickness crowned by hate.
A murder of Covid corvids,
perching on our humming lines,
watching for open windows,
swooping in
and stealing the breath of our people.

I invoke my sister crones,
daughters of the Goddess,
Mother Earth.
Ripe in our universal consciousness,
we emerge claiming our infinite power
to heal the disease and wounds of others
in this carnage.

As we dance to the music of our spirits
the mystery of our union with the Divine is revealed.
We move to the Truth within us,
circling the fire,
veils floating like wings of doves
behind us.

Alas, we are the healers,
ritually raising our vibrations
above the din of suffering.

We summon the clouds of corvids,
the great messengers beyond time and space
from the ether.
To them, we sing a song of Love,
transmuting death into Life.

Taking wing, they transport the energy of our message
to desperate souls in need,
altering their destinies.
An alchemical flight.

The raven whispers into their hearts,
to rid the land of Covid
the answer lies within.

*With tender unseen hands
we reach across the wasteland,
working with magical force
to lift the afflicted into the light
of curative restoration —
never to pass this way again.*

*We, the crones, have taken them
into their rite of passage
as the cycle of destruction ends
and we all live in freedom forever.*

MY DRAGON-WELL SWORD | JIANXUN GAO
(TRANSLATION BY JOCELYN ZHAO, REVISED BY DAWN LI)

Away from home in Xiamen
I can't enjoy the colors of Heron Island.
Daily I stare at bougainvillea.
At night, towards home, my thoughts roam.
How I wish my 3-foot Dragon Well Sword
could kill evil spirits and keep you whole.

I then went overseas.
While it is night for you, it is daytime for me.
Family and hometown are on the Wuhan frontline.
At the same hour every day I call you.
Write us more poetry, you say!
How can words relieve my longing for home?

EVOLVING | OLIVIA AVERY

*In the bloom of our youth
when we still thought we were immortal,
we did not glimpse how short time could be
before it runs out.*

*Earthly vigil is pressing in on us
as we face this sojourn together
against desolation and demise.*

*No boundaries.
We are on the brink
of the invisible, moving
dangerously to clutch us
in vice-like talons, spreading
extermination amongst us.*

*And legions of us are repulsed by deliberate, uncaring,
unmasked herds who appoint themselves judge and jury,
irreverently placing death sentences
on the remaining innocent.*

Embroiled

The masked bulwark
garners the horde of those who cultivate life
with fortitude,
facing the unseeable,
fixed to oppose the obstinate few
who are willing to risk life
for a few moments of pleasure.

And those weak are unmasked,
convinced they are valiant
as they swarm,
many self-selected to perish,
inwardly manifesting
the covert touch of deception.

But the robust, concealed inhabitants
push the unseen far away
never touched by it,
evolving out of chaos,
born of the cosmos,
the masses survive to thrive again.

POETS MAKING SPIRITUAL MEDICINE | RENHUI

our world is mourning
deadly coronavirus has spread
to every corner of the globe

Guanyin's compassionate
thousand arms and eyes
are not enough to stifle the blow

within weeks
Half a billion were on lockdown in China
migrant workers shriveled up in street corners
and wild animals are back on the roads

Infected States of America
fight about masks or no masks, reopening or closing
as seniors on ventilators gasp for breath
"10,000 more body bags please"

Embroiled

*now more Buddhas and heroes
have come forward—
doctors and nurses
guards and PPE makers
and hearse drivers*

*singers on Italian balconies
answering the battle cry
and poets on keyboards
making spiritual medicine
for the world!*

4 MOURNING

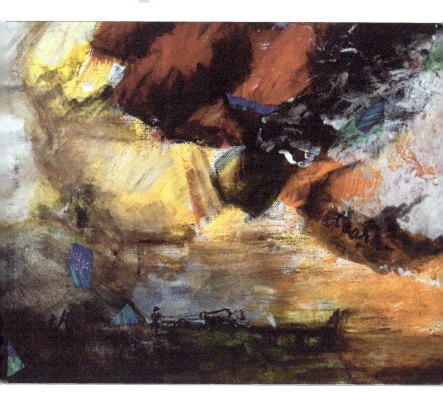

The wound is the place where the Light enters you.

— RUMI

SHOOTING STAR | JON WELSH

By the time I was visible,
I was gone. A goner.
I'm glad you saw me—
a miraculous moment,
witnessing my death.
Remember where you were
when you wished upon me.
Remember songs of hope
and loss; remember
trying to figure the mystery of my life,
its arc reflected in the dark sky
against your inner darkness.
Wish upon me now
that you will be the shooting star
others remember: live before you die.

BREATHE | JUDE-BRAIL UMAHI

quarantined midnight dawn unmasked
to bathe beneath warm rising sun;
dreamy dewdrops my lungs once asked
but ill denied to stifle fun...

locked up in ribcage starved without air,
twenty-four days of solitude;
battling to breathe amidst despair,
I gasped for hope and fortitude...

to stir up butterflies again
and dance with rosebuds as they bloom;
exhaling every breath of pain
to inhale petrichor's perfume...

most precious is this breath of life
to fight for in the face of fear,
and through all my weeks rife with strife
if I still breathe then you can dare...

ON PASSING | THANISHA SANTHOSH

When someone loses a dear one
we say we are sorry for their passing,

as if their husband has just moved
to the next town
and not died of a cardiac arrest,

and their daughter didn't kill herself
by overdosing on barbiturates.
Instead, she is simply,
right this moment,
on a train somewhere...

...upon a sequestered bridge
or asleep, perhaps,
under a field of lemon trees
as far as the eye can see.

*I think it is a lovely way to speak of someone's absence
without making their presence obsolete —
of sending time on a wild goose chase
in search of itself.*

*I wonder how many words we've invented
with the sole purpose of cushioning a blow?*

*Of pushing aside reality —
pithy and obstinate —
and leaving a small, bright space
for the pretty, rosy, illogical things
to go on existing?*

*What might be a softer way,
for me to use then, if i were to say,*
help me, i want to go on existing?

UNMASKED | FRANK LEIBOLD

her mask is off
teardrops everywhere
she's dressed for the ball
but he's not coming
the world is in despair

THE MAPLE | DEVON BROCK

*The maple is taller than yesterday,
peppered with birds and orange bloom — aloof
below an unscarred blue.*

*But that is the maple, those are the birds,
and that is the sky.*

*And though I cannot unsee
unfettered Spring, I cannot unsee
suspicion, the revulsion of hands,
breath and similar heats
that strain against our leanings.*

*I cannot unknow the slow drawn wind
and the shattered hope
clung brief in a tube.*

*Take to your pens, dear ones,
mark this time — scrawl that once
in a Spring not come, shriveled
and short of breath,
all Springs must take their measure.*

TIME FOR TEARS | PAULA GOODMAN

Tears need time,
rain needs space—
let them fall
with solemn grace.

If you're crying
you are living.
What you feel
is some grieving.

Where there is loss
and heartfelt sorrow,
there is a lesson
to learn tomorrow.

It doesn't matter
how you feel,
the sharpest pain
to you is real.

Mourning

*Confused, bewildered
out of place—
hurt, shocked—
hearts misplaced.*

*Allow the storm
to bring the tears.
It's ok—
they dissolve the fears.*

*Every raindrop
ever formed
needs a place
to be born.*

*After the storm
the crying is done.
Storm clouds part—
replaced by the sun.*

AT THE END OF APRIL | NIGEL de COSTA

It is a strange spring this year,
as one dreary day pulls after it another,
like a stream of silk handkerchiefs
conjured from a smiling magician's sleeve,
but look closely . . .
that smile's a grimace,
the silks are grubby cotton — monochrome, soiled,
yet flourished, as if something of wonder.

The sun, so fickle at this time,
today is brazen and bold,
browning grass whose green
is already a memory.
The languid heat, draining my will,
points to a summer of inactivity
and missed chances.

The camellia's magnificent pinks
and dazzling whites, once heralding a glorious year,
now lay shrivelled, trampled,
and, like our plans, left to rot.

Down by the river,
the rush of water around the weir
and the sound of its torrent
are a welcome contrast to the stillness elsewhere.

Mourning

This clears my mind,
like the audiobooks that I play during sleepless nights.
I listen to them but never really hear the words.

I stare listlessly at the water,
at the eddies and whorls
and calmer stretches,
where shoals of small fish
line up in tight formations
to fight the current
threatening to wash them away.

It seems an age since there was bustle
or anything that could be described as frenetic.
Time feels like a toy
lost in childhood,
now unexpectedly found,
puzzling in its familiarity and novelty,
leaving me bemused.

I steal a few moments on a park bench,
an illicit rest, a brief pause,
an opportunity to people-watch,
speculating how other lives might be lived,
wondering whether others feel
as alone as me.

HOPE BEYOND CORONA | JOHN FINKELSTEIN

Death lurks in the corridors,
lingers for that last gasping breath.
A woman's body motionless like a rock upon the sea,
soulless.

We didn't see coronavirus coming.

Before it arrived, dreams
were a bright yellow cork bobbing in the water.
Vibrant, alive, irrepressible.
A bird, its feathers protecting the soul.
Free to go to new places, unconfined.
Not locked down.
Life was good.

Yes there was fear — that's human.
But then, life as we knew it changed.
A bursting balloon.
Our dreams exploded.
Life hung in suspension.

Many spend their last lonely days in a hospital bed.
So many deaths and we tell ourselves,
"Things will be different.
There will be a new normal."
Isn't this simply re-calibrating hope?

Our very pores bleed hope.
Life and hope —
consecutive links in a precious chain.
But is this hope?
To live a good life and die
a peaceful or a horrid death?

A viral emptiness?
Or is there something more?
A hope of eternal life?
A body that doesn't age —
whose gasping breath does not signal final death?
Yet life goes on —
forever.

MY SIMPLE DREAM | ARCHIE HAYNES

I dream a simple dream
to fall asleep and rest and see
my loved ones close.
This prayer I cherish most.

I dream that virus vipers are no more
and grocery shelves are stocked galore,
where coughing's no harbinger of death,
and breathing's a joy with every breath.

I dream of shaking hands and trading smiles
not buying bread after driving miles,
nor returning home to wash and scrub
with soap and water and alcohol rub.

Mourning

*I dream of standing in a cheering crowd
not fearing I'll don a funeral shroud.
A dream where children play at school
and swim with friends in a backyard pool.*

*Still, this simple dream is far from true,
since more and more contract this flu,
and further countries shutter to survive
in hopes the day will come when they'll contrive*

*a simple hug, a smile, a kiss,
having escaped this deepening abyss.
A dreamworld free from fear and despair,
life returning to normal everywhere.*

TOROIDAL HEALING (FROM A TRINITY OF CIRCLES ~ 1ST RING) | RANDALL S.

A moment's time…
ushered a pause
in quavering uncertainties,
while conflicts
whispered confusion
from erratic winds.

The air began to tingle
with rising connections,
as unforgiven burdens
sought their release
in castaway shadows.

There,
floating in a morph of circles,
loving eyes lit with teardrops,
like divine fiber optics
in a sweep of measured rays,

upholding infinity—
 through patience,
  upon longsuffering;
   transferring, epiphanies
    with feeble handles
     for my shallow understanding.

Knowing our incessant need
 to caress soft blankets,
  thus, weaving it into us
   for tender healings.

So true revelations
 ripen seeds of mercy
  into final fruits,
   with a universal
    taste of salvation.

The moment time
 ushered a pause...

ENDURANCE | PAULA GOODMAN

Sometimes there are
no words to say
a soul in pain
will look away

When you lose
there is no smile
What's close to you
will sting a while

And when the final
curtain falls
dirt below
the surface calls

Remember though
the love that was there
and after death
you still can care

Keep holding on
and don't let go
This is the only
part I know

My friend, my dear
you had to leave
I cry my tears
into my sleeve

Mourning

When we let go
of agony
grief is good
because you loved me

And when I'm done
I'll dry my eyes
do my part
and realize

It always was
and meant to be
that I had you
and you had me

So beautiful
the time we had
I learned from you
what made me glad

And now apart
so physically
but in my heart
you'll always be

Cherished time
is assurance
for when apart
provides endurance

5 QUEST

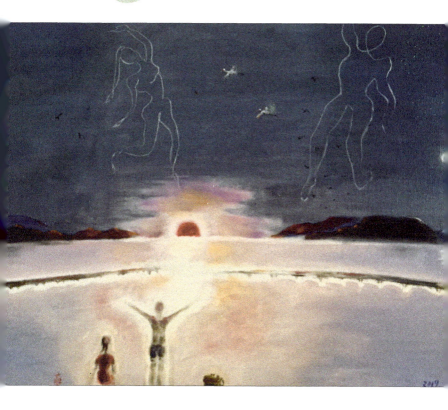

*First principle: never to let one's self be
beaten down by persons or by events.*
—MARIE CURIE

HUM | BRIJIT REED

in these garments
are the remnants
of meaning and memories,
adjacent to my flesh,
and to my bones.

embroidered within my heart,
this matrix is mine.
it records the shine
of each pearl I've cast away.

days devoted to earth and sky,
summoning spirits
with sweetgrass-scented prayers,
in escort of the tranquil snap of sparks
and the smoky, perfumed hope
that unites us with the clouds
and drinks from the sun.

elixir of the gods
pours from the stars
and nourishes the Earth
in arcing colors of refracted light,

Quest

*while humanity perches
on the sharp surface
of Occam's blade,
tempted by illusion,
but desirous of Truth.*

*we chase Maya's dreams
with the studied aerial navigation
and the stuttered flight
of a buttery, fluttery, butterfly
...fluttering by...*

*on paper-thin wings
but a heart full of life.*

*a forest of mirrors
reflecting our faces to eternity.
infinite options for Maya,
but only One unfurling reality
in a boundless continuum —
a hum,
of Now....*

THIS IS MY PRAYER | SARITA VERMA

In isolation,
we still have the birds and the moon,
stars and sunshine.
Trees sway in the spring, summer begins.
Wind chimes, chores, and children's games.
Unexpectedly, life tests you.
Together we come to fight this situation
and find solutions.
We have music and good times to think of
in the safe confines of our homes.
It's easier to live with the imperfections within.
Let's face the one outside full throttle,
flattening the curve.
In solidarity, we stand.
Let's spread the love and create some cheer.
Keep calm and behold the light within.
We'll send prayers to bring a safer tomorrow.
Peace be upon everyone.

HEALING IN THE WIND | JUDE-BRAIL UMAHI

an ashen whisper eclipses
this peccant sod,
exhaling that ominous
breath from hades'
lungs of woe and wrath...

upon this field trodden with
the guilt hatched
from the forbidden and
the hidden, to bend
brave knees and will to wilt...

and from the cusp of crypt's coma —
that slumber steep...
hiatus rose from heaven's
womb of mercy
with a blossom of solace...

waving dirgeful twilight away
to herald new dawn
sharing flowers fragranced
with hope and healing
across the breadth of grieving land...

HEAL YOUR WOUNDS |
ROWAN VANSKYVER KILLIAN

Heal the wounds that hide within —
the ones that hide in the blood and attack all in existence.
But don't worry.
These wounds are nowhere, except for —
well, just about everywhere.
These tiny little wounds may cause space to tremble itself
unless we come together to fix the world.
To heal, we all must contribute our efforts to eliminate
these wounds.
And what will we get?
Relief.
Much of the craziness in the world will be relieved
if we all come together and solve this one true problem.
For now, we all must hide in this little shell away from
all else
and this seems to go on forever.
If we all contribute and make sacrifices,
our wounds will heal.

PAIN | MIAO XI
(TRANSLATION BY WILLIAM GONG, REVISED BY DAWN LI)

Flowers may vary,
but only in colors and shapes.
When life fades,
let a smile send it away.

Dignity or life,
who can say which has more weight?
When desires are rampant,
dignity is speechless
and naked corpses become silent.

Humans or animals
endure the same death and soul.
Whether or not we reincarnate,
let us drop anger and hate.

Let love
fill this void of our world.
Let the soul rest in peace,
whether we are human or deity.

Life may be different
but who is not afraid of pain?
When our body turns into smoke in the cremator,
from that moment,
don't ask to be saved!

A STRING OF HOPE | MYTHRI ARJUN

like a string of hope
little ones clapping hands and tapping feet

listening to the music of the past
sad tunes turn joyful with their smiles

I joined them in their fun, their hugs
bad days forgotten, left behind

holding to truth, dear, let's step forward
a new horizon joined with the light of dawn

new skies to travel under and with time,
silence, to speak once again, in person

unwinding the tangled strings that reach high
like a kite to fly far above all our troubles

THE SPARROW'S SONG | MJ DONNELLY

*I literally took them for granted
most of my life, these one-ounce minstrels
until recently
when I heard them, really heard them
for the first time*

*singing joyfully like the first day of creation
as though they hadn't a care in the world!*

*Disputing the sorrowful spirits
gleefully proclaiming their unwavering
optimism*

*heralding sunrise, offering lyrical canticles
to the dawn, aware of mankind's
faults and folly, but celebrating a new day
nonetheless, with hope...*

AS SOLDIERS OF TOGETHERNESS, WE WIN! | JON VON ERB

All events,
great or small, joyful or of crisis in nature,
exhibit a purpose.
As far as mankind is concerned, it is how we,
the human race,
deal with what this life has dealt us
that makes the difference.
That we've been taken by surprise is a given;
mankind's ingenuity
opens our doors to inventiveness.

Facing Covid-19 presents a call for responsibility.
After 4 months, we know the dangers,
the risks to be taken or ignored,
the outcomes, and the results of each choice
we have been given.
Acting NOW is the key that secures the lock
on our preservation.

Everything,
living or merely existing
has a shelf-life;
eventually,
all living organisms will die or disappear
into the mist of nonexistence.
As guardians of our keep as a people,
each of us must delve deep into our conscience.
When we do all we can to protect ourselves,
the protection of others around us will be steadfast.
No virus can live (exist) without a host —
no vulnerable hosts = no existing virus —
plain and simple.

Positive thoughts and action are our weapons.
Complacency must not enter this battlefield.
We must render this crisis extinct.
With unselfishness and fortitude
as our shields,
we can, and we will, end this blight,
but only
ALL TOGETHER!!

ROOTED | BRIJIT REED

I cannot see your feet
beneath the table
so I do not know
if they've taken root
in the soil,
casting branches
like inverted trees
deep into the earth.

if they have,
I know that you are nourished
by the light that kisses your face,
the rain that washes you clean,
and the clouds
that provide the shade
that cools your skin
as they sail across the sky.

if they have,
I know that you are the grass
that softly waves hello
to the poppies and sunflowers
that grow in the meadows
in ribbons of red
and banners of yellow.

if they have, I know that you sing
with the voice of every bird
and hum with every bee,
whistling through the hollows and caves
in whispered thoughts of love and devotion
to the creatures sheltered by them.

if they have,
I know that you are the stars
spangling the sky,
cradling the moon,
and casting a silver glow
on everything below.

if they have,
I know that you are the mothers
that rock your babies,
the fathers that wipe away the tears,
and the children who dance in the fields
as their cells multiply
and grow them tall and strong
into the mothers and fathers
who rock their babies
and wipe away their tears.

*if they have,
I know that the Earth
breathes with your every breath,
pulsing with Life
whether you wake or slumber,
in dreams, Truth, or stillness.*

*if they have
or have not,
I know that Life is Present
in the beginning,
and the middle,
and the end.*

THE TRUE SELF | PATRICIA ROOKS

The True Self is never offended
if the ego has been transcended.
For humor with love having blended,
all anger and viciousness is mended.

CIRCLES OF HARMONY | RENHUI

Life is full of confusing shapes
until we've learned to
draw circles
from within ourselves —
our own life force

Each of us is an energetic system
affecting and affected by those around us
our health depends on
the balance of yin-yang principles
and the harmony of the five elements
metal, wood, water, fire, and earth
within us and surrounding us

Within us plays the alchemy of the elements
Around us performs the symphony
of collective battles and triumph

The good doctor is wise
who knows you and herself
She does not let your symptoms trick you
To cure you of any disease
she finds the root cause
and teaches you to self-heal

Quest

You will become a doctor yourself
because your body
is your gift and your carrier
Your lifestyle, emotions, and thoughts
are more important than your pills

Be still
Listen to your body as the body never lies
Open the gateways
Harmonize the elements
Charge up the energy channels —
Those meridian rivers that run through your organs
connect
connect the water in you
connect the fire in you
connect the earth in you

Draw circles every morning
Invite joy and love into your circles
No more anger and anxiety
Life is not an accident
There are no accidents

Those are not mistakes
Go with the flow
Begin your dance

Dance to the music
that moves you
Dance in sacred circles
of harmony
When harmony is achieved
the body will heal itself

Dance dance dance

BIRD'S-EYE VIEW FROM UNDER AN OAK TREE | QIHONG (RICHARD) WANG

In this autumn afternoon,
I sit alone under an old oak tree.

An unnamed bird keeps screaming among the treetops,
I don't know if it is singing happiness,
complaining of sadness,
or telling its stories of life.

Beside me is a pair of white butterflies,
slowly flying back and forth,
doing the present dance of their lives—
Don't they worry about tomorrow?

In the glow of this Sunday in the fall,
I look far into the promise of the dawn of the world,
reflecting on the day after tomorrow
and tomorrow.

6 EMERGING

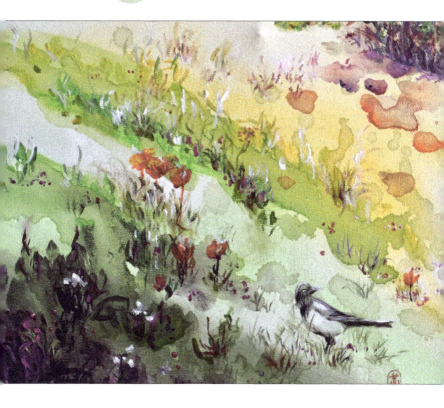

*Suffering in search of truth gives
true meaning to the truth.*
— EGYPTIAN PROVERB

NEST | DEVON BROCK

If the moon
is not dragged through night
by dogs, I will twist the ropes
and make it so. I'll strap mules
to the sun and plow — cut
deep and cumulus furrows,
seed rain and turn my vast mouth
to the sea. Whereupon,
I will spit the whale and breach.
All things are of my making.
If in every beginning
is a word, then the word
must be Love. A symphony
of snakes is born of this,
this coiled hiss. And if not,
I will make it so.
There is no rift I cannot flood
with the wave of a hand, a word —
no cleave or condescension
that is not swept away.
It is your turn now, your turn
to speak the world into being —
your turn to make
a basket of your hands
and see what nests there.

DANCE AGAIN | JUDE-BRAIL UMAHI

this unseen hex that vexed our souls
and stirred this storm within
sneezing around, breeding death tolls
eclipsing dream and grin

calm now provoked fear to evoke
drowning our livelihood
this evil yoke made grown men broke
and dampened the merry mood...

frustrating as this war may be
still, fight we must all fight
dawn will herald that crystal sea
after this cursed twilight

shed your worries, don't be sorry
nor let them weigh you down
this too will pass in a hurry
from uptown to downtown...

and once more we will dance again
embracing without fear
like rainbow after summer rain
hopeful without despair...

FELLOWSHIP | FRANK LEIBOLD

When this heartbreak finally ends
We'll break the stale and stifled air
With cheer and tidings greeted
Brisk the smile and crisp the hand
Extended quick for shaking
Those sparkled eyes and sunny faces
Make for two cheerful spirits indeed
Two strangers each offering greeting
In a pleasant bond of fellowship meeting

THERE IS HOPE | AURUM DI ANGELO

Pain, Darkness.
Bleak silence.
You almost want to give up on life.

Busy days
are easy to get through
but these quiet nights
are the ones that test you.

You lie down tired,
shutting sleepless eyes,
finally making peace
in the silence of a fading night.

You hear chirping birds.
They make you smile.
You open your eyes
and turn to your side.

Earth's sun reaches out,
lending you its brightness,
suggesting, "You
must never give up!"

Reminding you
that after every dark night,
there is always
a bright new day!

HERE AND NOW | THANISHA SANTHOSH

When all of this ends,
footfall will greet the pavement
like rain pattering on grey tarmac.
The street inundated, no discrimination,
with patent leather work shoes
or tattered rubber boots or light-up floaters (size 4).
Not a single child will complain
about early morning school timings
or the ominous weight of backpacks
on their nimble shoulders.

School buses will ply once again,
their tires screeching, ferrying skittish children
in the height of pubescent glory,
absolutely vigorous and mildly displeased
that the world didn't end,
no, not this time.
Young lovers, however,
will be the only species to remain indoors,
having found a common bed to copulate, like hermit crabs.

It will take one week for everybody
to start complaining about the traffic again,
but for now, mile-long traffic jams will be
no less delightful than a date at the teahouse or
an opera concert.

Emerging

*Street vendors will never be more garrulous,
hawking rotund mangoes and spiny pineapples
 and wind up toy cars
and cucumbers and big balloons in fluorescent colours
with small balloons within them and sweetmeats and
sunglasses and pencils with strawberry-scented
erasers fitted
into their tops.*

*The gregarious call of the street urchin,
once menacing nuisance, will now
be mellifluous symphony,
collecting in the ear horns of drivers everywhere.
For once, journey will supersede destination—
we have waited for months, they will say,
what is an hour or two in a stagnant sea
of motor cars?*

*When all of this ends,
children will go back to looking each other
in the eye again
and adults will go back to looking away—
unless in search of loquacious companionship
or a good bar fight.*

*A heroin fiend will make his way
to an unknown park bench armed with
spoon and silver foil,
jonesing for his first fix after months
of going cold turkey.
Somewhere an abused woman will return
to her abuser, no less virulent
than the virus,
only this time she won't be saved.
Elsewhere a grieving woman will return
to therapy
only to ask her therapist,*
and how are you today?

*The skeptics will refuse
to take their masks off for another month,
suspicious as ever of their government's
machinations and so it won't be very rare,
in a microcosm of naked mouths,
to spot one covered in surgical blue.
Grandchild will never again miss
an opportunity to huddle close to grandparent—
or at least remember
to telephone on their birthdays.*

Emerging

The monsoons will come and with them
new problems, new conflicts, new headlines;
a nuclear threat will plague a powerful nation,
a suicide bomber will decide to detonate
in a train full of people,
another ethnicity will be discreetly cleansed in a camp
but the world will refuse to concentrate.

Another species, perhaps toothcarps
or carpet sharks or green sea turtles
will move from the endangered list
to the extinct one.
A country's farmers will perish
in dysentery and drought
and women everywhere continue to languish
for equal wages,
but we will argue this year that our eyes
have grown too heavy to bat.

There will be newer accidents to celebrate
and fresher corpses to mourn,
when all of this ends
it is not to say suffering will.
Suffering knows no end.

*Suffering will never end
but today will
and so will tomorrow and the day
after that,
and so long as each day ends,
melting into the interface of the next,
we will trust the sun to rise again
and we will learn to breathe once more
then
and tomorrow
and here
and now.*

THIS MOMENT AFTER COVID | JAYANTEE KHARE

this moment after Covid
some affirmations to amend
some paths to bend
some ties to mend
some relations to tend

this moment after Covid
some pictures to crop
some attachments to drop
some trends to stop
some corners to mop

this moment after Covid
some memories to delete
some acts to repeat
some fears to beat
some targets to meet

this moment after Covid
some issues to deal
some wounds to heal
some moments to steal
some emotions to feel

WINGS OF FAITH | JUDE-BRAIL UMAHI

faith found me amidst doubt and fear
lifting me from ashes of pain
denuding me from the despair
that drove my weary soul insane

faith set my feet on the path of hope
and with each step healing was paved
along the odd road he helped me cope
and my soul he led to be saved

faith perched upon my breath to breathe
to inhale the free gift of air
denied another grave a wreath
and treated me kindly and fair

faith gifted me the will to live
became the wind beneath my wings
because of him I soared to thrive
like a butterfly whose flutter sings...

THERE'S A SEED FOR EVERY SORROW | FAY BALLERINO

There's a seed for every sorrow; take your pain, let it grow.
Nurture your hurt; don't be afraid to reap what you sow.
Water it with your tears, plant it gently in a sunny row.
Let it live in your heart till it sprouts roots in your soul.
Maybe nothing changes today, perhaps not tomorrow,
but with time and patience, one day you will know —
the best grounds for growth are sprinkled with woe.
Pain has blossomed into beauty; you are more than whole.

A FLIGHT OF FANCY | PHOENIX ARADIA

Come walk with me down to the bridge —
the one past the nurse's station.
Let's do it now, before the doctors return —
to hell with our medication.

We'll feast on the nectar from honeysuckle,
pick some blackberries along the way.
We'll go down to the water's edge,
and write our names in the clay.

Once we're there we can strip off these gowns,
and reclaim our true identities.
We'll stand naked beneath the nourishing sun,
and bask in our new found amity.

Emerging

You'll say my name to the west winds,
and to the east I'll say yours.
When the two collide in this place,
the wind will howl and roar.

Then we'll walk to the edge of the bridge
and we'll clasp each other's hands.
We'll jump into the river below,
wiggle our toes in the sand.

Now we two wild-eyed creatures
are free to roam again at last—
never again to be bound and dressed
by the judgements of the past.

WITH THE HELP OF FAITH IN THE AFTERMATH OF COVID-19 | JON VON ERB

We, those left behind,
must trust that death is yet a guided glide
into the next realm of creation.
Death is but a step of continuance in the cycle of
existences.

The cocoon becomes the butterfly.
The butterfly, in dying, welcomes
a new beginning.
That beginning dusts back into the earth,
which in turn,
nourishes the next generation
of new life entities.

Lovingly, we miss
those who once stood beside us,
yet with the gracious passing of time,
we feel
those who have passed into the next domain
on the winds of today.

Emerging

*In the eyes of our children
we see
all things growing,
their expressions,
their smiles —
all fly in our memories
through our inner eye.*

*We realize the magnitude of life.
What a special
gift it is to be alive
and we promise ourselves
to make each and every moment
a joyous continuum of those we love.*

*The spirits of those
who have left us urge us
onward in the glory
of their lights'
aura.*

RISE | JUDE-BRAIL UMAHI

fear may come up with that story
of faith fading before our eyes
yet we'll rewrite our own history
that amidst ashes hope will rise

trodden upon like common dirt
trampled beneath boots of despair
still we will rise like a desert
stirring sandstorms in the air

we may be weak but not broken
our knees may bow but not our will
we'll wear courage like a token
and rise to face each odd and ill

we've cried enough — it's time to rise
take off the sackcloth of sadness
dry our tears and wipe our eyes
we'll rise, robed once more, in gladness

Emerging

like springtime we will sprout again
from frozen ground buried in snow
and let the rain wash every pain
we'll shine once more like a rainbow

then we'll rise again and banter so
as fear and caution take flight
kindle the flame of hope to glow
let nature's beauty grace our sight

we'll make sense of what normal was
our new normal we will embrace
with grateful sigh surrounding us
we'll rise to claim our place

ACKNOWLEDGMENTS

THIS BOOK WAS NOT possible without the generous support of many poets from all over the world, many of whom are published on allpoetry.com. We express our deep appreciation for Kevin Watt who founded allpoetry.com in 1999 and nurtured many poets from all over the world for several decades.

We also want to thank Brijit Reed for collecting many poems from poetic circles beyond allpoetry.com. She is the editor of this book and contributed two of her own poems to this effort.

The illustrator, Yanfang, generously offered her art works to the project. She is not only a talented painter, but a poet herself!

Many people have devoted their time and energy to the development of this book. Their names are listed in the Key Contributors section.

Finally, we would like to thank Susan Shankin for her dedication and professionalism as a creative director and publisher. She has been with us from the very start and has gone far above and beyond in her duties to help turn an idea into a beautiful book.

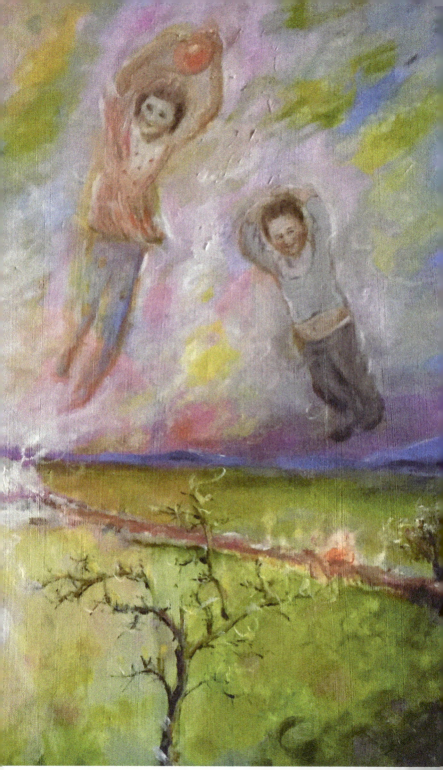

KEY CONTRIBUTORS

MANAGING EDITOR: DAWN LI, PH.D. (USA)

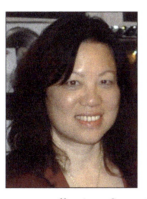

Dawn Li (Renhui) is an entrepreneur, poet, and educator. Having lived and worked extensively both in the US and China, she has embraced a life philosophy that centers on the human ideals of collaboration and collective advancement. Many of those experiences are chronicled in her poetry collection, *Song of a Lotus Leaf,* published in early 2020 by Precocity Press. Her doctorate dissertation on T. S. Eliot reveals insights hidden in his modern poetic masterpieces through the perspective of death and enlightenment during a cultural crisis. Seeing poetry as a powerful healing tool, she organized like-minded poets on allpoetry.com and beyond to contribute to the creation of healing poems, which became this poetic medicine project in support of our fight against Covid-19. Dawn is the head of a data analytics firm and has taught college level courses from culture to computer science. She holds a doctorate in American Literature and a master's in information technology from George Washington University. (poeticmedicinebook.com, allpoetry.com/renhui)

ILLUSTRATOR: YANFANG, PH.D. (FRANCE)

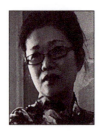

Yanfang (Jun Li) arrived in France as a Chinese student in the early 1990s. She now teaches in the Department of Cross-Culture and Language Studies at the University of Paris. A passionate and prolific painter, she was inspired by the artistic atmosphere in Paris and deeply influenced by Western Modernism, including the works of the Impressionists and Expressionists. She enjoys merging Western artistic styles with both Chinese spirit and techniques. Her work depicts both past and present, forms and abstract transformation. Her paintings range from watercolor to oil painting, acrylic, and Chinese ink painting, and illustrates both narrative and colorful form. She has developed her own artistic expression, transcending borders and established styles. She is widely invited to exhibit her work in France and has recently begun to show it in other countries, including China and Italy, as well. All the artworks in this book are Yanfang's original creations. (instagram.com/xiaoyanartist)

EDITOR: BRIJIT REED (USA)

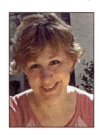

Brijit is an author, screenwriter, editor, ghostwriter, and freelance writer. She's comfortable writing in a variety of mediums, genres, voices, and tones — everything from historical epic to biography, light comedy, and science — but she especially loves poetry, history, culture, philosophy, spirituality, and self-help. She's particularly drawn to complicated material and loves learning new things, often conducting research for her own projects, as well as for those of her clients. In addition to her freelance work, she's currently writing a book on the topic of peace. (brijitreed.com)

ASSOCIATE EDITOR: PAULA GOODMAN (CANADA)

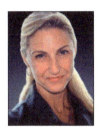

Paula is a deep thinker and as a writer, she enjoys sharing her words. She's passionate about working to motivate, inspire, empower, and provoke thinking. She believes that we are all here for a reason. Paula's professional experience is disbursed across various leadership roles in service industries. It is through battles in life that she discovered the birthright of dignity. She has written several hundred poems and many of her poems are viral with hundreds of likes and comments. She is known as the "Word Jedi Poetess" on Linkedin. (linkedin.com/in/paulagoodman1)

ASSOCIATE EDITOR: JON VON ERB (USA)

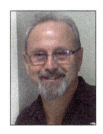

Jon is a poet and editor who mentors poets worldwide online and lives in Southern California with his husband of 45 years. Professionally, he practices therapeutic and medical massage therapy. His first career was that of a ballet dancer, choreographer, and professor of classical dance techniques in America and Europe. Alternatively, he has been a floral designer and has taught literature and fine arts in his hometown of San Francisco. He loves dogs, nature, positivity, and thought-provoking ideas, which he trusts is reflected in his poetry. November 2019 marked the date of his first published book of poetry, *Insights of a Dancing Poet*. (allpoetry.com/jon_the_von)

ASSOCIATE EDITOR: JUDE-BRAIL UMAHI (NIGERIA)

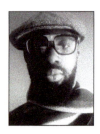

Call me an aesthete by nature; but never a snob. I am a soul divinely blessed with besprinkling quill to waltz wonderfully woven words from hues and emotions into poetry for the bliss and beauty of humanity. (allpoetry.com/judd)

ASSOCIATE EDITOR: FRANK LEIBOLD, PH.D. (USA)

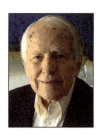

Frank was born in Brooklyn, NY, and raised in Pittsburgh, PA. He earned his engineering degree from the University of Dayton, his MBA at the University of Pittsburg, and his PhD at the age of 54, at the University of South Carolina. Married with four children, he has ten grandkids living in Virginia. He has worked as Assistant Dean, Professor & Chair of the marketing department at Averett University, President of Alcatel N.A. Company, General Manager and Corporate Director of Technology Development at Corning Incorporated, and numerous other management positions over the years. Frank is also an acclaimed author. His first book, *The Key to Job Success in Any Career: Developing Six Competencies That Close America's Global Skills Gap* (2010), was about America's global skills gap. He's a mentor to entrepreneures and small businesses, and currently, he's also an aspiring poet. His poetry style is minimalist with a pyramid-formatting structure. (allpoetry.com/docfrank)

COORDINATOR: YASMEEN MCGETTRICK (USA)

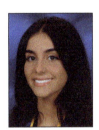

Yasmeen recently graduated from the University of California, Santa Barbara, with a Bachelor of Arts in French. She is multilingual and extremely passionate about languages. In addition to working for Data and Analytic Solutions (DAS), she serves as a consultant and French translator for the World Bank Group. Yasmeen has greatly enjoyed working on *Poetic Medicine in the Time of Pandemic* with Dr. Li and the rest of the team.

COORDINATOR: JOCELYN ZHAO (CHINA)

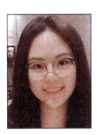

Jocelyn (Xiaoqing) is an international student in the United States, currently majoring in Analytics (MS) at American University. Her bachelor's degree was in interpersonal and organizational communication from George Mason University. She loves to coordinate events where people gather to share learning and life experiences and enjoys gardening and hiking.

BIOGRAPHIES

Phoenix Aradia (USA) was born in Bradenton, Florida, and eventually made her way back to Florida after living in Tennessee, New York City, and Pennsylvania. Depression and mental health issues have been her unwelcome companion for many years. She writes to connect with others and hopefully, occasionally inspires and intrigues them as well. She currently lives in Tampa, where she enjoys frequent thunderstorms, beaches, and the company of her family—especially her 9-year-old son, Fox, and her many animal friends (twitter.com/phoenixaradiaa, allpoetry.com/phoenix_aradia).

Mythri Arjun (India) published in the *Rewrite Sunlight* anthology. She loves to write about nature and life. (allpoetry.com/mythri_arjun)

Olivia Avery (USA) is 75 years old and lives in Los Angeles. She's the mother of two adult children and one hilarious cat. Although she's never previously submitted anything for publication, she was inspired by the theme of this project. Until now, Olivia has only written poetry as a way of thinking out loud and for her own personal enjoyment.

Fay Ballerino (USA) is a young poet who's passionate about sharing her expressions of beauty and sincerity, whether that be through her writings or other creative outlets, such as the musical and visual arts. This is her first published work, but she hopes to continue refining her perceptions through the medium of poetry. (instagram/fayballerino; allpoetry.com/fay_b)

BOBBIE BREDEN (USA) is a retired lady leatherneck, renaissance woman, and lover of life's mysteries. (allpoetry.com/captain_b2)

DEVON BROCK (USA) is an aging punk who left the city for the sticks to discover that all things large can be found in a greasy cardboard box under the passenger seat of a junked out pickup truck. His work has appeared in *La Piccioletta Barca*. (sweetandbittergreens.com)

PAUL BROTHERS' (USA) poetic interests started in the 60s. Later, as a sports blogger in the Boston Globe's Newspaper/Website, he decided to start writing 24-line postgame wrap-up poems about the Boston Celtics game that was just played. He continued writing postgame poetry for over 12 seasons. He became an "institution," as he was the first to blog each game-ending follow-up story with its poetic rendition. With Covid-19, sports largely stopped, and he joined allpoetry.com. (allpoetry.com/paulbrot)

BRIAN CARLIN (Scotland) lives in Girvan, Ayrshire, Scotland, and writes poetry because he's the only translator he knows for the wordless thoughts in his head. (theprimate.wordpress.com)

Essama Chiba (Egypt) is a poet, author, and content editor from Egypt, as well as a member of International Poetry Fellowship. She has been published in over twenty poetry anthologies worldwide and co-authored several poetry books. She received a certificate from Global Poetry Planet Organisation for best poem of the year in 2018 for her poem, "Bitter Harvest." Since leaving her career in broadcasting, she is now co-hosting a poetry podcast on Blogtalkradio. She was married to Abed Al Kader Naguib, a TV director and scriptwriter, and shared over forty drama series for many television stations with him in the Arab world. (allpoetry.com/essama_chiba)

Cecelia Cran (UK) lives in Kegworth, North West Leicestershire, United Kingdom. She's 73 years old, married, and has a daughter, son, and four grandchildren. She's interested in local history, and has connections with her local Heritage Centre. Some of her poems have been published in other publications. She has also had poems included in several collections after attending poetry workshops. Her poetry is varied and she writes on a wide variety of themes, but has particular interests in expressing herself through poems about wartime and conservation. (allpoetry.com/cecelia_cran)

Nigel de Costa (UK) is a new poet living in the UK with his three children. Poetry is something he's been interested in for many years but has only tried his hand at writing it recently and he's discovered that it's something he enjoys very much! (allpoetry.com/stig-ndc)

AURUM DI ANGELO (India) is a medical student from India. She is an avid reader and amateur writer. She has been writing since age 12 and has written many poems for her school magazines throughout her middle school and high school years. A few years ago she began to write on allpoetry.com. Writing has healed her and helped her grow through tough times. Her words are a reflection of what she feels, and she hopes that in her poems, her readers find hope too. (allpoetry.com/aurum_di_angelo)

MICHAEL J. DONNELLY's (USA) education in writing consists of a few college semester hours of technical and creative writing as part of a non-commissioned officer development course taken years ago while he was an active-duty member of the Army. He has been published in a few anthologies through allpoetry.com groups and has a web page entitled, *Musings from a Northern Latitude*. (mikejoedonnelly57anchak.wordpress.com)

KIM ESCOBAR (USA) attended Antioch College and worked as a chef for many years. More recently, writing has become her passion. She has been published in several anthologies and will be included in an upcoming magazine as well.

PENG (GARY) FANG (USA) is a New York licensed attorney. He has published over 60 scholarly articles in newspapers and peer-reviewed international journals. His translated legal documents were edited into books and published internationally. Gary has been reported on TV and by newspapers. In addition, he has written many poems and published some of them in China.

JOHN FINKELSTEIN (Australia) is married with three grandchildren and loves writing poetry about human nature (especially family), nature, and spiritual issues. Previously unpublished, he enjoys that his writing can affect the emotions of others. (allpoetry.com/john_l indsey)

SHARON FLYNN (USA) has been published in a number of anthologies and small press poetry journals such as *Lucidity*, *Parnassus Literary Journal*, and *Midwest Poetry Review*. She is the author of her own collection of poetry, *Dance With The Brazen Moon*, which was a result of a poetry book contract awarded at a poetry convention in Philadelphia. She continues to be inspired to create new poems. (allpoetry.com/ivyrose)

JIANXUN GAO (China) was born in April 1969 in Dawu, Hubei, China. He is a Professor and Director of the Human Resources Department at the university in Wuhan. His studies primarily involved higher education management, but also various publications, including *Legends of the Qin and Han Dynasties*, *Research on Higher Education*, and over fifty academic papers. He was depressed during the early stages of the epidemic but was later deeply moved by the courage of the number of heroes who rushed in to rescue the citizens of Wuhan. This astonishing contrast motivated him to praise the spirit of kindness and share positive messages with the warm and inspiring words of his poetry.

GREG GAUL (USA) was an advertising executive and had clients worldwide for nearly fifty years. His poetry has been in print in anthologies and poetry journals. He has done readings for poetry groups and on radio. His works appear on poetrysoup.com, allpoetry.com, and poemhunter.com. (allpoetry.com/greg_gaul)

PAULA GOODMAN: see bio in Key Contributors section

ANNA-MARIA HARTNER (Germany) is an epidemiologist with an interest in infectious and zoonotic diseases who holds a Bachelor of Arts in public health from Johns Hopkins University. A lifelong writer, Anna-Maria's primary work is in health communications, but she has a passion for writing poetry on subjects outside of her field—especially those that reference her joy of nature. When not reading, Anna-Maria loves baking pastries, climbing mountains, and maintaining her indoor garden. She currently resides in Germany among family and several dogs.

ARCHIE HAYNES (USA) writes poetry to focus his thoughts and experience presence. He finds comfort in poetic expression and writes to articulate his inner experience of the world. As a psychotherapist, he is privileged to have others share themselves with him and works to alleviate their psychological suffering. His poems are an attempt to honor our efforts to accept life as it unfolds. (allpoetry.com/archie_hay)

Norbert James (USA) is 61 years young and has been an unpublished poet for 45 years, but his writing has been loved and cherished by those he's been blessed to share his musings with. He is honored to be published in this fine compilation of poems that historically documents this once-in-a-lifetime pandemic. Of German-Polish ancestry, Norbert tries to live a life of spirituality and love. He hopes his few words included in this book will show that he is just one of many who share a love for all of mankind as we all strive to survive this pandemic.

Jayantee Khare (India) is a post graduate in mechanical engineering by qualification, teacher by profession, and a poet by passion. A native of Bhopal, she settled in Pune, is a light worker (Reiki master), and writes poetry in English and Hindi. She has been writing since childhood. She collects the words from her inner self and writes them all down. (jugnuwrites.blogspot.com, instagram.com/writerjugnu)

Rowan Vanskyver Killian (USA) is a 9-year-old poet from Venice, California. He originally started writing about random things and eventually came up with titles in a small notebook. His poems flow from these titles and send the reader into his world. This is his first publication.

Caren Krutsinger (USA) publishes her work at allpoetry.com. She believes that she is a puppet to her whims and imagination and is on earth to bring joy and love. She enjoys learning new ways to express herself and share soul-self with readers. (allpoetry.com/pinkfaerie5)

FRANK LEIBOLD: see bio in Key Contributors section

DEBRA SUE LYNN (USA) has been published locally and around the United States and the United Kingdom. She has been writing poetry since the 1980s and performing her works around the country at open mic shows at various clubs, including the Green Parrot, in Key West, Florida. She has been invited to read her work in cafes in Providence, RI, St Louis, MO, and in California. She self-published a book of poetry entitled *Tales from the Heart* which she performed at Barnes and Nobles in Daytona Beach, FL, followed by a book-signing. Debra Sue is seen as a professional storyteller and poet in Florida and lives on the water in a cozy, eclectic condo on the east coast of that state, where she enjoys her privacy and quietude. (allpoetry.com/liquidmindforever)

GLENN MERRILEES (Scotland) has been published in 22 poetry anthology books as well as several booklets to date, and has been invited twice to the Scottish Parliament to read his mental health awareness work. (allpoetry.com/glenn_merrilees)

HENRIQUE FORMIGONI MORAIS (Brazil) was born in Sao Paulo, Brazil, where he's lived all his life. He is currently an undergraduate student in philosophy and wishes to pursue a career as a researcher in that field. He dreams of being a professional writer as well, and eventually wants to write novels and publish his own collection of poetry.

Poetic Medicine is his first time as a published writer (and, ironically, not in his first language). (reddit.com/user/strangeglaringeye)

Carmela Patterson-Mooney (USA) now 79, grew up in West Philadelphia. She has published over 10k poems on allpoetry.com and has over 1200 followers. She has a wonderful family with five children, 13 grandchildren and seven great-grandkids. Carmela graduated nursing school at 47. She was a coronary critical care nurse at Crozer-Chester Medical Center until retiring in the late '90s. After her husband passed away, Carmela mourned, then built a good but different life. She volunteered with the Legion of Mary, providing Bible study and fellowship to men incarcerated at a local prison. She met Gary Mooney and was married again on Valentine's Day in 2020. (allpoetry.com/patterson-mooney)

Brijit Reed: see bio in Key Contributors section

Renhui (Dawn Li): see bio in Key Contributors section

Patricia Rooks (USA) is 83 years old and has been a teacher all of her adult life. She has worked 20 years in the classroom teaching, 29 years as director of religious education in parish situations, and ten years tutoring GED and ESL students, while working for a refugee resettlement program as well. She self-published ten small children's books as her jubilee project. She lives in assisted housing and writes for her own enjoyment. (allpoetry.com/Patricia67)

RANDALL S (USA) is the author of *The Lyrical Odyssey of Sifter (the Dream Collector)*. His poetry book tells the adventures of a dream collector written in rhyming quatrains. Other characters include a cosmic cowboy as a rainbow collector, Chaos as god of whirlwinds, and the dream collector's sidekick, Sketch Buddha. (allpotery.com/randall_s)

THANISHA SANTHOSH (India) best describes herself as a poet that attends medical school. She writes because it's the only way she knows how to breathe — by stringing words like beads through a loop. She's currently studying to be a psychiatrist and is the doting dog mother of two. She likes to read, travel off the beaten path, cook, and paint botanical illustrations in her free time. (instagram.com/thanishaa, theministryofmotheatenmulberries.wordpress.com)

ROBERT STONE (USA) is a New Jersey native who learned to write before he learned to bleed. Poetry is his manic side, the scatterbrain allowed to run rampant. The wordplay, the rhythms, the paintings — they are all routes for him to explain his madness, to wrap it in words so others can say, "You too?" Previously, his work has been published by *The Altar Collective*, an independent magazine originally based in Los Angeles. (instagram.com/linesofstone)

JUDE-BRAIL UMAHI: see bio in Key Contributors section

ALFRED VASSALLO (England) was born in Sliema, Malta in 1956, and established himself as a lover of literature and arts. Besides acting and directing, Freddie wrote a series of programs for Radio Malta, in his teens. At the age of fourteen, he started writing poems in his language, and in later years, he wrote many plays in English and self-published his poems in several books. Poetry cures his soul. (alfredvassallo.com)

Sarita Verma (India) lives in Pune, India and has been sharing her work at hellopoetry.com since December 2016. She's also published a book of poetry, *Thoughts & Words*. (facebook.com/saritaaditya.verma.3)

Jon Von Erb: see bio in Key Contributors section

Qihong (Richard) Wang (China) was a reporter and editor for Xinhua News Agency back in China before he came to the US to pursue his graduate degrees. He has been a banker for many years but writing poetry has been his passion since he was in junior high school. He published his first poems in the *College Weekly* when he was studying at Wuhan University. These days he doesn't write very often, but each of his poems illustrates his feelings and thoughts about life. He publishes his poems in Chinese magazines and newspapers in the US, as well as on social media platforms.

Jon Welsh (USA) has published two volumes of poetry, *Beatitudes and Holy Rollers,* and *Reversal is The Way,* which has been published in *Lost Lake Folk Opera* and *The Fresno News*. For several years, he also published the political blog, *Democratic Views*. He has read his poetry in Washington, DC, Chicago, IL, Nashville, TN, and Tblisi, Georgia. He credits the University of Chicago, the Library of Congress, and American University for his formative experiences. Today he travels mostly in his imagination.

MICHAEL MCGIBNEY WHELAN (USA) published *After God*, in 2014 and it tells the story of his life-long lover's quarrel with God. His collection of poems on the famed late Irish poet and novelist, Dermot Healy, was featured in *Éirways* magazine. *Clay Feet* was included in the *Martin Stannard* August 2013 collection, featured on *The Best American Poetry* blog. Whelan won first prize in the juried Leitrim Guardian 2012 Literary Awards. His work has appeared in *The Wallace Stevens Journal, The Innisfree Poetry Journal, The Coachella Review, The Healing Muse, Little Patuxent Review,* and *The Galway Review*. (michaelwhelanpoetry.com)

MIAO XI (China) was born in Hunyuan County, Datong City, Shanxi Province, China, and grew up there. She's an official poet for China National Geographic Poetry and a signed columnist for China's largest online tourist magazine, *Wanjingtai*. She's also the Development Director of North American Love Poetry Society and a member of The Datong Writer's Association. Many of her works have been published in various Chinese newspapers and other media. Living in a mountainous area has greatly kindled her passion for writing poetry and she believes that life's greatest glory is to purify oneself and illuminate the path for others. (wechat ID: hssmx1970)

YANFANG (Jun Li): see bio in Key Contributors section

For more information, visit poeticmedicinebook.com

Lightning Source UK Ltd.
Milton Keynes UK
UKHW050244201220
375215UK00004BA/249/J